CRITICAL CARE
BEDSIDE REFERENCE

CRITICAL CARE BEDSIDE REFERENCE

WENDY SWOPE ACNP-C

iUniverse, Inc.
Bloomington

Critical Care Bedside Reference

iUniverse books may be ordered through booksellers or by contacting:

iUniverse
1663 Liberty Drive
Bloomington, IN 47403
www.iuniverse.com
1-800-Authors (1-800-288-4677)

ISBN: 978-1-4620-2919-8 (pbk)
ISBN: 978-1-4620-2920-4 (ebk)

Printed in the United States of America

iUniverse rev. date: 07/11/2011

2011

WENDY
SWOPE
ACNP-C

CRITICAL CARE
BEDSIDE REFERENCE

No discussion - Just facts | Swope

"When you are up to your ass in alligators it is difficult to remind yourself your initial objective was to drain the swamp"

Unknown

Contents

1
Electrolyte Replacement

Potassium Replacement Protocol
(normal = 3.5-5.1 meq/L)

SERUM POTASSIUM LEVEL	TOTAL POTASSIUM REPLACEMENT
3.5-3.7 meq/L	KcL 20 meq IVPB
3.2-3.4 meq/L	KcL 40 meq IVPB
2.7-3.1 meq/L	KcL 60 meq IVPB
2.3-2.7 meq/L	KcL 80 meq IVPB
< 2.3 meq/L	KcL 80 meq IVPB and contact provider

Repeat potassium level
2 hours after the infusion is complete.
Correct as indicated above.

Magnesium Replacement Protocol
(normal = 1.6-2.3 mg/dL)

CORRECTED MAGNESIUM LEVEL	TOTAL MAGNESIUM REPLACEMENT
1.5-1.9 mg/dL	2 g $MgSO_4$ IVPB
1.2-1.4 mg/dL	4 g $MgSO_4$ IVPB
0.8-1.1 mg/dL	6 g $MgSO_4$ IVPB
<0.8 mg/dL	8 g $MgSO_4$ IVPB and contact ordering provider

Corrected Serum Mg =
Mg x 0.42 + 0.05 (4 - albumin in g/dL)
Repeat serum Magnesium level
2 hours after infusion complete.

Phosphorus Replacement Protocol
(normal = 2.4-4.5 mg/dL)

3 mmol of potassium phosphate = 4.4 meq of potassium

- Pharmacy will mix $NaPO_4$ or KPO_4 in 250cc NS
- Use **KPO_4** if K is **less than 4.0 mEq/L**
- Use **$NaPO_4$** if K is **greater than 4.0 mEq/L** and **Na is less than 145 mEq/L**
- Infuse over **4 to 6 hours**
- Repeat phosphorus level 6 hours after infusion is complete

CURRENT PHOSPHORUS LEVEL	TOTAL PHOSPHORUS REPLACEMENT
2.0-2.5 mg/dL	15 mmol K or Na phosphate IVPB
1.6-1.9 mg/dL	30 mmol K or Na phosphate IVPB
< 1.6 mg/dL	30 mmol K or Na phosphate IVPB and contact provider

Calcium Replacement Protocol
(normal 8.4-10.2 mg/dL)

Corrected Serum Calcium =
Calcium + (0.8)(4 - albumin in g/dL)

**Repeat ionized calcium level 2 hours
after infusion complete**

IONIZED CALCIUM LEVEL	CORRECTED CALCIUM LEVEL	TOTAL CALCIUM REPLACEMENT
3.5-3.9 mg/dL	7.8-8.3 mg/dL	2 grams Ca Gluconate IVPB
3.0-3.4 mg/dL	7.0-7.7 mg/dL	4 grams Ca Gluconate IVPB
<2.9 mg/dL	<6.9 mg/dL	6 grams Ca Gluconate IVPB and contact ordering provider

Insulin Protocol - Sliding Scale
Using regular or rapid acting insulin

1. **Very low schedule (Insulin-sensitive)**
   1. BG 150-199: 0.5 unit bolus Insulin
   2. BG 200-249: 1 units bolus Insulin
   3. BG 250-299: 1.5 units bolus Insulin
   4. BG 300-349: 2 units bolus Insulin
   5. BG Over 350: 2.5 units bolus Insulin

2. **Low schedule**
   1. BG 150-199: 1 unit bolus Insulin
   2. BG 200-249: 2 units bolus Insulin
   3. BG 250-299: 3 units bolus Insulin
   4. BG 300-349: 4 units bolus Insulin
   5. BG Over 350: 5 units bolus Insulin

3. **Medium schedule**
   1. BG 150-199: 2 unit bolus Insulin
   2. BG 200-249: 3 units bolus Insulin
   3. BG 250-299: 5 units bolus Insulin
   4. BG 300-349: 7 units bolus Insulin
   5. BG Over 350: 8 units bolus Insulin

4. **High schedule (Insulin-resistant)**
   1. BG 150-199: 3 unit bolus Insulin
   2. BG 200-249: 4 units bolus Insulin
   3. BG 250-299: 7 units bolus Insulin
   4. BG 300-349: 10 units bolus Insulin
   5. BG Over 350: 12 units bolus Insulin

Insulin protocol: gtt

Blood Sugar Goal

Medical and Surgical ICU patients - BS range 90-140

Acute MI (or ACS) patients - BS range 125-200

Medical and Surgical patients - BS range 100-200

Check BS Q 1 hr until BS in range x 2 hrs, then Q 2 hrs x 4, then, if stable, Q 4 hrs.

If BS > 250 after four insulin drip changes, notify provider.

Insulin drip titration: May use this initially or when BS changes > 75 mg/dl/hr.

After 1-2 hours:

BS increasing or unchanged - Increase rate 50-100%

BS decreasing by 75-100 mg/dl/hr but > goal - Maintain drip at same rate

BS decreasing by 100-150 mg/dl/hr - Decrease rate 25-50 %

BS decreasing by > 150 mg/dl/hr - Decrease rate 50-75% Hold drip 1 hr **only** if BS < 250

BS within goal, continue drip at current rate and check BS Q 1 hr x 2 then Q 2 hrs x 4.

Insulin Drip Titration: May use this when BS changes are < 75 mg/dl/hr.

BS > goal - Increase rate 0.5-2 units/hr.

BS 80 - 100 mg/dl/hr - Decrease rate 0.5-1 unit/hr.

BS > 60 - 80 mg/dl/hr - Hold drip 1 hr, then decrease rate 0.5-2 units/hr.

BS < 60 mg/dl/hr - Give 100 ml D_{10} or 200 ml D_5W When BS > 100 start drip at 0.5-2 units/hr less than the previous rate.

If sensitive to change in rate use lower end of change (0.5 units/hr). If insulin resistant use higher end (2.0 units/hr).

Converting from Insulin gtt to bolus dosing

Calculate the total units of insulin used over the last 6 hours and multiply by 4 for the 24 hour usage.

Multiply this number by 0.8 for the estimated subcutaneous basal insulin requirements using glargine insulin.

Insulin gtt used per 6 hours x 4 = Total insulin used
Total insulin used x 0.8 = Glargine insulin dose daily.

"Medicine, to produce health, has to examine disease."
Plutarch

2

Comparison Charts

Steroid potency/conversion chart

Drug	Equivalent Pharmacologic Dose (mg)	Mineralo-Corticoid Potency	Biological Half-Life (hrs)
Hydrocortisone	20	2+	8-12
Cortisone	25	2+	8-12
Prednisone	5	1+	24-36
Methylprednisolone	4	0-0.5+	24-36
Dexamethasone	0.75	0	36-54

Relative Selectivity of Sympathomimetic Agents for Adrenergic Receptors

Agent	A1	A2	B1	B2	DA
Dopamine	0 to +++	+	++	+	+++
Norepinephrine	+++	+++	+++	0	0
Epinephrine	+++	+++	+++	++	0
Isoproterenol	0	0	+++	+++	0
Dobutamine	+	0	++	+	0
Milrinone	0	0	0	0	0
Phenylephrine	+++	++	0	0	0

Relative Potencies of Vasodilator Agents

Agent	Arterial Dilation	Venous Dilation	PCWP	SVR	CO	HR
Phentolamine	+++	+	-	--	++	+
Nitroprusside	+++	++	--	---	++	-/+
Nitroglycerin	++	+++	--	-	+	-/+
Hydralazine	+++	-/+	-	--	-/+	+

*"Educating the mind without educating
the heart is no education at all"*
Aristotle

3

Arterial Blood Gas and Acid Base Disturbances

pH
Acidosis <———— 7.35-7.45 ————>Alkalosis

Respiratory
Alkalosis <———— CO_2 35-45 ————> Acidosis

Metabolic
Acidosis <———— HCO_3 22-26 ————> Alkalosis

	Acid	Normal	Alkalotic
pH	< 7.35	7.35-7.45	>7.45
PaCo2	>45	35-45	<35
HC03	<22	22-26	>26

Example:

pH is 7.49 (alkalotic) - CO2 is 48 (acid) - bicarb is 37 (alkalotic).

Since there are two alkalotic results, this gas reflects a metabolic alkalosis.

Anion Gap Calculation

A calculation of the anion gap is used to identify the cause of metabolic acidosis.

$$\mathbf{AG} = (Na^+) - (Cl^- + HCO_3^-)$$
(A normal anion gap is 8-12)

Causes of an elevated anion gap

Acidosis Present	Acidosis Absent
A MUDPILE **A**lcohol **M**ethanol **U**remia **D**iabetic ketoacidosis **P**araldehyde **I**ron/ **I**soniazid **L**actic acidosis **E**thylene glycol	Dehydration Alkalosis Sodium salts of unmeasured anions Antibiotics Decrease in unmeasured cations

Osmol Gap Calculation

Osmol Gap =
measured serum osmolality − calculated osmolality
Calculated osmolality =
2 x (Na mmol/L) + (glucose mmol/L) + (urea mmol/L)

Clinical Conditions that Cause Acid-Base Disturbances

Anion Gap Metabolic Acidosis	Non-Anion Gap Metabolic Acidosis
Analgesics Cyanide Carbon monoxide Arsenic, Alcoholic ketoacidosis Toluene Methanol Metformin Uremia Diabetic ketoacidosis Paraldehyde Phenformin Iron Isoniazid	Volume contraction Excess Bartter's syndrome Post-hypercapnic alkalosis Hypokalemia Alkali ingestion/infusion glucocorticoids or mineralocorticoids

Respiratory acidosis	Respiratory Alkalosis
Central nervous system de-pression Pleural disease Lung disease Acute airway obstruction Neuromuscular disorders Thoracic cage injury Ventilator dysfunction	Toxins CNS disease High altitude Severe anemia Pregnancy Lung disease/hypoxia Anxiety Cirrhosis of the liver Fever

A **lactate level** may also be ordered to help detect and evaluate the severity of hypoxia and lactic acidosis. Although a significantly elevated lactate level indicates increased anaerobic metabolism, the test is neither specific nor sensitive for hypoperfusion. The test may be performed on either arterial or venous blood samples.

Lactate Reference Range

arterial: 0.36 - 1.25 venous: 0.90 - 1.70

"The life so short, the craft so long to learn"
Hippocrates

4
Neurological

Glasgow Coma Scale

Motor Response
6 - Obeys commands
5 - Localizes to noxious stimuli
4 - Withdraws from noxious stimuli
3 - Abnormal flexion
2 - Extensor response
1 - No response

Verbal Response
5 - Alert and Oriented
4 - Confused, yet coherent, speech
3 - Inappropriate words and insensible phrases
2 - Incomprehensible sounds
1 - No sounds or intubated

Eye Opening
4 - Spontaneous eye opening
3 - Eyes open to speech
2 - Eyes open to pain
1 - No eye opening

The score is a total of one number from each section

Sedation and paralysis

Indications
fear and/or anxiety
control of agitation
facilitation of mechanical ventilation/airway management
amnesia during neuromuscular blockade

Levels of Sedation
Minimal: At this level the patient is able to protect their airway and is able to respond to verbal commands.

Moderate: This may also be referred to as conscious sedation. The patient is still able to respond to verbal command and it able to protect their airway. They have depressed consciousness with the medication provided.

Deep: The patient can respond to stimuli only after vigorous stimuli. They may not be able to protect their airway and may need an artificial airway.

General anesthesia: At this level the patient is not arousable to stimuli. The patient's airway is compromised and an artificial airway and mechanical ventilation is generally required.

Sedation Scales
There are many sedation scales in use; all have the goal of being able to safely monitor the efficacy and comfort of the patient while procedures or treatments are performed. The Ramsay Sedation Scale is a representative of this goal.

The scale used and the level of sedation desired is to be determined by the ordering provider

Ramsay Sedation Scale

Score   Response
1. Awake - anxious, agitated, restless
2. Awake - calm, cooperative, oriented
3. Asleep - brisk response to loud auditory stimulus
4. Asleep - sluggish respond to loud auditory stimulus
5. No response to loud auditory stimulus but responds to painful stimulus
6. Does not respond to painful stimulus

Sedation Medications

Drug	Loading dose	Maintenance dose
Dexmedetomidine	1 mcg/kg over 10 minutes	0.2-0.7 mcg/kg/hr
Midazolam	0.1-0.3mg/kg	0.03-0.25mg/kg/h
Lorazepam	0.03-0.07mg/kg	0.03-0.07mg/kg at 4-6h intervals
Propofol	0.5-2.0mg/kg	1.0-6.0mg/kg/h
Ketamine	0.5-1.0mg/kg	1.2-6.0mg/kg/h
Haloperidol	5-10mg	repeat dose every 2-4h

These agents may be used in conjunction with narcotic agents either in bolus or gtt form for pain management.

Paralytic Medications

Indications

Treatment of symptomatic hypercapnia
Treatment of symptomatic hypoxemia
Airway protection against aspiration

Drug	Bolus doses for intubation	Doses for continuous infusion
Succinylcholine *do not use if elevated potassium*	1-2 mg/kg	N/A
Etomidate	0.3 mg/kg	N/A
Vecuronium	0.2 mg/kg	0.8-1.2 µcg/kg/min
Atracurium	0.5 mg/kg	5-10 µcg/kg/min
Cisatracurium	0.2 mg/kg	1-10 µcg/kg/min
Pancuronium	Do not use	1-2 µcg/kg/min
Mivacurium	0.25 mg/kg	1-15 µcg/kg/min
Rocuronium	1 mg/kg	4-16 µcg/kg/min

Used in Rapid Sequence Intubation protocols

Monitoring Paralytic Efficacy

Train of four: used during use of continuous infusion of neuromuscular blocking agents

Electrical stimuli are periodically applied to either the radial nerve or the facial nerve at the temporal region. If there is no neuromuscular blockade the nerve twitch will be brisk and consistent. With blockade present there will be a reduction in number of twitches as well as briskness.

Medically Induced Coma

Indication
Typically used in the case of traumatic brain injury in order to reduce the activity of the brain to assist in reducing swelling.

Coma Medications

Drug	Dose
Pentobarbitol	Induction 5-10 mg/kg over 1-2 hours, then 1-3 mg/kg/hr
Thiopental	Induction 5 mg/kg over 1-2 hours, then 2.5-5 mg/kg/hr

Efficacy of this medication regimen may be based on continuous EEG monitoring with the goal of burst suppression.

Intercranial Pressure Monitoring

Indication

Used to monitor intercranial pressure (ICP) and make treatment decisions in the case of traumatic brain injury. A drainage system may also be used to allow excess CSF and/or blood to be released from the cranial vault.

Normally, the ICP ranges from 5 to 15 mm Hg.
ICP's > 20 may be life threatening and are usually treated.

ICP waveform

ICP monitoring waveform has a flow of 3 upstrokes in one wave.

P1 = (percussion wave) represents arterial pulsation
P2 = (tidal wave) represents intracranial compliance
P3 = (dicrotic wave) represents aortic valve closure

In normal ICP waveform P1 should have the highest upstroke, P2 in between and P3 should show the lowest upstroke.

On the monitor, if P2 is higher than P1 - it indicates intracranial hypertension.

Treatment Considerations in TBI

Treatment decisions in traumatic brain injury involve careful consideration of all body systems. Hypoxia is avoided and generally so is hyper-oxygenation.

Hypothermia may be considered, along with paralytics, to reduce the oxygen requirement of the brain.
Adequate blood pressure must be maintained in order to ensure perfusion to the brain.

Cerebral Perfusion Pressure (CPP) = Mean Arterial Pressure (MAP) - Intracranial Pressure (ICP)
CPP=MAP-ICP

The goal is a target CPP of 50 to 70 mm Hg

Cushing's triad
This is an ominous finding that is an indication of increased intercranial pressure and possible impending brain herniation.

Cushings Triad consists of hypertension (systolic), bradycardia and widening pulse pressure (rising systolic, declining diastolic).

"He who has health, has hope;
and he who has hope, has everything"
Arabian Proverb

5

Respiratory

Oxygenation is the process by which concentrations of oxygen increase within tissue

Ventilation is the mechanical process that moves air in and out of the lungs.

Respiratory Failure is defined by either failure to oxygenate or failure to ventilate

Failure to Oxygenate

This deficit most often occurs where the pulmonary capillary and alveolar surface meet. It is caused by:

1. Diffusion defects wherein the alveoli are perfused but are not ventilated.
2. Shunt, wherein the alveoli are ventilated but not perfused.
3. There are degrees of these conditions and both may be present at the same time.

Failure to Ventilate

This deficit is typically caused by mechanical obstruction such as pulmonary emboli or mucous plugging. This condition results in reduced alveolar ventilation and a resultant increase in the PaCO2 > 50 mmHg.

Types of Oxygen Therapy

Nasal cannula can provide flows ranging from 0 to 8 L/ min, and a maximum of 40% O2 delivered.

Simple Mask can provide flow rates of 10L/min and a maximum FIO2 of 55%

Non-rebreather can deliver 10-15 L min and a maximum FIO2 of 80%.

Mechanical ventilation can deliver a maximum FIO2 of 100%

Mechanical ventilation

Common indications for use:

- Acute lung injury
- Apnea with respiratory arrest
- Chronic obstructive pulmonary disease
- Increased work of breathing
- Hypoxemia with PaO_2 with supplemental $FiO_2 <$ 55 mm Hg
- Neurological disease syndromes

Intubation Procedure

A mnemonic for performing Rapid Sequence Intubation (RSI) the 7 Ps

1. Preparation - prepare all necessary equipment, drugs and back-up plans
2. Preoxygenation - with 100% oxygen
3. Premedication - with a sedative
4. Paralyze - using an appropriate paralytic
5. Pass the tube - through the vocal cords
6. Proof of placement - using a reliable confirmation method
7. Post intubation care - secure the tube, ventilate

Post intubation care will also include: elevation of the head of the bed and scheduled and prn oral care to reduce oral bacteria and resulting ventilator associated pneumonia.

Acute respiratory distress syndrome (ARDS)

This syndrome causes a decrease is lung compliance making it difficult for the lung to inflate as well as deflate adequately. The decrease in compliance makes oxygenation problematic resulting in hypoxemia refractory to increased supplemental oxygen.

ARDS may be precipitated by lung injury caused by sepsis, trauma, or severe pulmonary infections.

ARDS is characterized by dyspnea, profound hypoxemia, decreased lung compliance, and diffuse bilateral infiltrates on chest radiography.

Critical Care Bedside Reference

ARDS is considered with acute onset of:
1. PaO2/FiO2 ≤ 300 (corrected for altitude)
2. Bilateral infiltrates consistent with pulmonary edema
3. No clinical evidence of left atrial hypertension

Goal of therapy
Pa02 55-80 mm HG
Plat ≤ 30 cm H20
Vt 6 mL/kg predicted body weight (PBW)
PH >7.15

Predicted body weight calculation (PBW)
Males = 50 + 2.3 x (height - 60]
Females = 45.5 + 2.3 x (height - 60)

Initial Management of ARDS

1. The ventilator is initiated on Assist-Control mode. Settings should be made to achieve initial V_T = 6-8 ml/kg PBW (predicted body weight)

2. Set initial respiratory rate to 12-14 bpm.

3. Initial Fi02 of 1.0

4. PEEP is started at 5 mm and increased to achieve a Plateau Pressure of ≤30

23

Terms

Peak Inspiratory Pressure (PIP): The peak pressure exerted against the patients airway during the breath, this may be increased in the case of mechanical obstruction in the airway, lung or chest wall.

Peak Expiratory Pressure (PEEP): The airway pressure kept above atmospheric pressure at the end of the expiratory cycle on the ventilator. This also takes into account the airway resistance caused by the endotracheal tube.

Auto PEEP: The patient is initiating breaths out of sync with the ventilator causing stacked breaths. This situation creates an inadequate expiratory time.

Modes of mechanical ventilator support

Pressure cycled modes

Pressure Support Ventilation (PSV) The ventilator sets the RR, Ve and inspiratory time. Breaths are triggered by the patient's inhalation and limited by the set pressure.

Pressure Control Ventilation (PCV) The ventilator sets the inspiratory time. Breaths are triggered by the patient and the inspiratory time is determined by the ventilator

CPAP (continuous positive airway pressure) The patient initiates their own breaths and the machine provides positive pressure on the inspiratory cycle.

BiPAP is CPAP with pressure support at 5-20 cm H2O

Volume cycled modes

Control: The patient breathes in accordance with the ventilator at a set rate. The patient cannot add breaths.

Assist: The patient provides all breaths and the ventilator provides a preset tidal volume for these.

Assist/Control: As in Assist mode. If the patient's RR fall below a preset value - the vent then switches to control mode and provides the required breaths.

Intermittent Mandatory Ventilation (IMV) The vent provides the patient with a set number of breaths. The patient can initiate breaths and they are not supported with a fixed volume. The ventilator will deliver the set breaths even if the patient is exhaling.

Synchronous Intermittent Mandatory Ventilation (SIMV) provides supplemental breaths for the patient as needed which are synchronized with the patients inspiratory effort.

Spontaneous Breathing Trial (SBT) This may be used to determine suitability for discontinuing mechanical ventilation. It can be done by:

1. Putting the patient on minimum pressure support and PEEP.
2. Place the patient on CPAP.
3. Place the patient on a T-piece.

The patient would be placed on one of these maneuvers and observed for respiratory distress over a period of several hours.

Criteria for SBT

    VE < 15

    PEEP < 5.0

    FIO2 < 0.5

    F/VT < 105

    Gag/Cough Present

    Hemodynamically Stable

    Minimal secretions

    Cooperative

Criteria for Terminating SBT.

    Sat $\leq$ 89%

    HR Change $\geq$ 15 BPM and / or > 110

    SBP Change > 15mm Hg

    RR $\geq$ 35 BPM

    Signs of Patient Distress

Mechanical Ventilation trouble shooting

Problem	Possible causes
High peak and plateau pressures	Pulmonary edema, consolidation, atelectasis, mainstem intubation, tension pneumothorax, chest wall constriction
Increased difference between peak and plateau pressure	Bronchospasm, secretions, inspiratory circuit obstruction
Auto-peep	Insufficient flow rate or expiratory time, expiratory circuit obstruction, AC circuit with agitated patient
Low exhaled volumes	Circuit or cuff leak, insufficient flow rate, bronchopleural fistula
Increased respiratory rate	Change in clinical status, low tidal volume, insufficient flow rate or set ventilatory rate
High exhaled volumes	Inline nebulizer therapy
High minute ventilation	Hyper ventilation, hypermetabolism ,inefficient ventilation

A-a O2 Gradient

The A-a 02 gradient is calculated by measuring the gradient between alveolar and arterial PO2

$$\text{A-a gradient} = P_A O_2 - P_a O_2$$

Normal Gradient Estimate = (Age/4) + 4
Normal <1mmHg

The A-a gradient can be used to determine is the hypoxemia is a result of intrapulmonary or extrapulmonary causes.

An elevated A-a gradient, taking into account the Normal Gradient Estimate, may be caused by a defect in diffusion, V/Q mismatch, or right-to-left shunt.

Causes of Hypoxemia

With elevated A-a gradient
V/Q Mismatch
Shunt
Alveolar Hypoventilation

With Normal A-a gradient
Hypoventilation
Low FiO2

*"The only way to keep your health is to eat what you
don't want, drink what you don't like,
and do what you'd rather not."*
Mark Twain

6
Cardiovascular

Normal Hemodynamic Parameters - Adult

Mean Arterial Pressure (MAP): 70-90mm Hg
Central Venous Pressure (CVP): 2-8mm Hg
Pulmonary Artery Systolic Pressure (PAS): 20-30mm Hg
Pulmonary Artery Diastolic Pressure (PAD): 6-12mmHg
Pulmonary Artery Mean Pressure (PCWP): 6-12mm Hg
Cardiac Output (CO): 4-8 L/min
Cardiac Index (CI): 2.5-4 L/min.
Coronary Artery Perfusion Pressure (CPP): 60-80 mmHg
Stroke Volume (SV): 60-130 ml
Stroke Volume Index (SVI): 40-50 ml/m2
Systemic Vascular Resistance (SVR): 800-1200 dynes
Systemic Vascular Resistance Index (SVRI): 2000-2400 dynes
Pulmonary Vascular Resistance (PVR): 150-300 dynes

Determinants of cardiac output:

The cardiac output is the product of the stroke volume and the pulse rate. **CO = SV x HR**

Cardiovascular Definitions

Contractility is the innate ability of cardiac muscle to contract. This is not dependent on preload or afterload, also known an inotropy.

Preload is the measured amount of blood volume stretching the left ventricle as it fills. Venous return is the determinant for this measurement.

1. Venous return, therefore preload, can be increased by increasing circulating blood volume by adding fluids. It can be reduced by the use of diuretics.
2. Preload, not circulating blood volume, can be varied by the adoption of a head-down or head-up posture.
3. The effects of preload can be altered by the use of vasoconstrictor or vasodilator therapy on venous return.

Afterload is the pressure against which the ventricle must contract. Afterload for the left ventricle is determined by aortic pressure, afterload for the right ventricle it is determined by pulmonary artery pressure.

Afterload can be affected by systemic vascular resistance (SVR) or the pulmonary vascular resistance (PVR). This can be altered either by medications that reduce the tone of the arterioles (such as nifedipine and nicardipine) or by reducing blood viscosity.

Medication Notes

Positive inotropes, increase contractility and therefore increase the cardiac output.

Negative inotropes have the opposite effect, decreasing contractility and cardiac output.

Chronotropes change the heart rate by affecting the nerves controlling the heart, or by changing the rhythm produced by the sinoatrial node. **Positive chronotropes** increase heart rate; **negative chronotropes** decrease heart rate.

Hypertensive Emergencies

Category	Systolic		Diastolic
Normal	Less than 120	*And*	Less than 80
Prehypertension	120-139	*Or*	80-89
High blood pressure			
Stage 1	140-159	*Or*	90-99
Stage 2	160 or higher	*Or*	100 or higher

A **hypertensive emergency** is hypertension that is adversely impacting an organ system such as CNS, cardiovascular or renal. If left untreated this can lead to permanent end-organ damage.

Malignant hypertension is a sudden and rapid development of extremely high blood pressure. The diastolic blood pressure reading is often above 130 mmHg. This condition is typically genetic in nature.

The **goal of treatment** is to reduce the blood pressure steadily rather than abruptly. Consideration must be made of the patient's normal blood pressure, too quick a drop in blood pressure can lead to end-organ ischemia. **Therefore the initial goal of therapy is to reduce the mean arterial pressure by approximately 25% over the first 1-2 hours.**

Shock is defined as inadequate tissue oxygenation and perfusion as result of a sudden drop in blood flow through the body.

Treatment of shock

In all cases definitive treatment is dependent on the cause of the shock. Initial goals are to maintain hemodynamic stability through the use of fluids, vasopressors or vasodilators, ensure adequate circulating blood volume and management of oxygenation.

Hypovolemic: caused by a profound loss of circulating blood volume, either hemorrhagic or non-hemorrhagic. Characterized by a decrease in intravascular volume.

Cardiogenic: caused by damage to the heart and resultant decreased perfusion to end-organs. This may be myopathic, mechanical or arrythmic in origin. Arrythmias may be common and signs of heart failure are present.

Obstructive: caused by mechanical obstruction preventing adequate perfusion to the tissues. Pulmonary embolism is an example.

Distributive: caused by massive systemic vaso-dilation as a result of infection (sepsis), anaphylaxis or neurological damage

"Medicine makes people ill, mathematics makes them sad, theology makes them sinful"
Martin Luther

7
Renal

Causes of Acute Renal Failure

Prerenal azotemia
decreased extracellular fluid volume
gastrointestinal losses
burns
hemorrhagic hypotension
decreased effective volume
cardiac failure
cirrhosis/ascites
positive pressure ventilation
third spaced fluids
soft tissue trauma
hypoalbuminemia

Intrinsic azotemia
Glomerular disease
Interstitial nephritis
Vascular disease
Acute tubular necrosis (ATN)

Postrenal azotemia
Anatomic obstruction
Neurogenic bladder

Characteristics of Renal Disease

Marker	Prerenal azotemia	Intrinsic azotemia	Postrenal azotemia
Urine specific gravity	>1.020	1.012	1.012
Urine osmolarity (Mosm/L)	>400	300 ± 20	300 ± 40
Urine/plasma osmolarity	>1.5	1	1
Urine sodium (mEq/L)	<20	>30	<30
Fractional excretion of sodium (FeNa)	<1%	>1%`	<1%
BUN:Cr	20	10	10-20
Urine/plasma creatinine	>40	<20	<20

Diagnostic micro

Diagnosis	Urine sediment
Prerenal azotemia	Normal or near normal (hyaline casts and rare granular casts)
Postrenal azotemia	Normal or can have hematuria, pyuria and crystals
Intrinsic azotemia	See below
Glomerular disease	RBC, RBC and granular casts; abundant proteinuria
Interstitial nephritis	Pyuria, WBC casts, eosinophils and eosiniphilic casts
Vascular disease	Eosinophils
Acute tubular necrosis	Pigmented granular casts, renal tubular epithelial cells and granular casts

Action of diuretics

Loop diuretics: act in the thick ascending limb of the loop of Henle. They remove potassium, sodium and water.

Thiazide-type diuretics: act in the distal tubule and connecting segment. They remove potassium, sodium and water. They also cause an increase in serum uric acid.

Potassium-sparing diuretics: act in the aldosterone-sensitive principal cells in the cortical collecting tubule. They remove sodium and water while preserving potassium.

Dialysis

Acute indications:

- Metabolic acidosis not correctable with sodium bicarbonate replacement
- Life threatening electrolyte abnormality
- Acute poisoning with a dialysable drug.
- Fluid overload not expected to respond adequately to treatment with diuretics.
- Severe complications of uremia.

Chronic indications:

- Symptomatic renal failure
- Low glomerular filtration rate (GFR < 10-15)
- Difficulty in medically controlling fluid overload and electrolytes with low GFR.

Dialysis and filtration can be performed either intermittently or continuously. Continuous therapy (CRRT) is used for acute renal failure in the hospital setting. Due to the slow blood removal it is better tolerated by hemodynamically challenged patients. All forms of dialysis, except peritoneal, require vascular access.

> *"Be careful about reading health books.*
> *You may die of a misprint"*
> *Mark Twain*

8
Metabolic Derangements

Hypokalemia (< 3.5 mmol/L) is generally a result of substantial potassium losses as in prolonged emesis and diarrhea. May also be caused by decreased intake or as a side effect of medications.

Oral potassium supplementation is the preferred treatment method. If the potassium level is less than 2.5 mEq/L, intravenous potassium is given via slow gtt. Consider magnesium replacement also if that level is <2.0 mEq/L.

Hyperkalemia (>5.5 mmol/L) most often seen as a result of renal dysfunction causing decreased potassium excretion. May also occur in the case of significant cell death as this releases potassium into the bloodstream.

Treatment is dependent on the cause of the hyperkalemia. Glucose and insulin help push potassium from the extracellular space back into the cells. Sodium bicarbonate may be considered to correct acidosis and diuretics may be used to increase potassium excretion in the urine. Dialysis may be needed if these methods fail and renal failure is present.

Hyponatremia (< 135 mmol) is most often as a result of over ingestion of free water or hypotonic solutions.

It is important to correctly determine the fluid volume status in relation to the hyponatremia. This may be determined by an assessment of serum osmolality, urine osmolality and urine Na+.

Serum Osmolality

$(2 \times (Na + K)) + (BUN / 2.8) + (glucose / 18)$.
Normal Range = 285-295 mOsm/kg

Urine osmolality

Normal Range is 500-800 mOsm

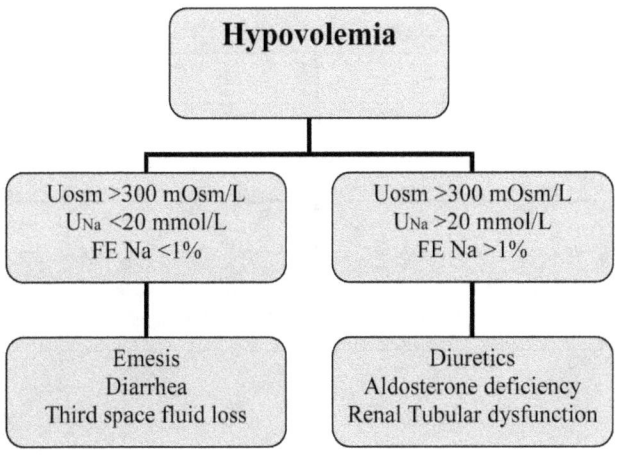

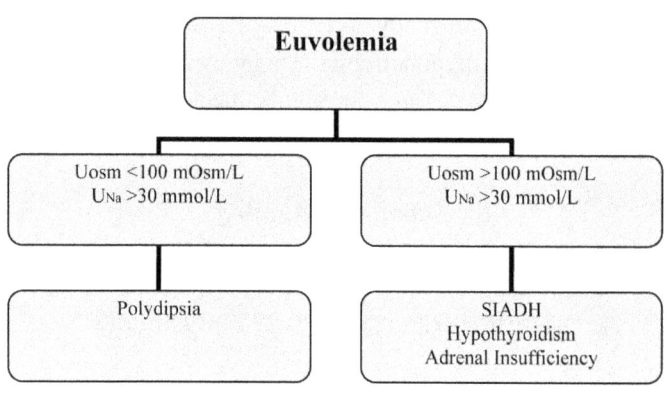

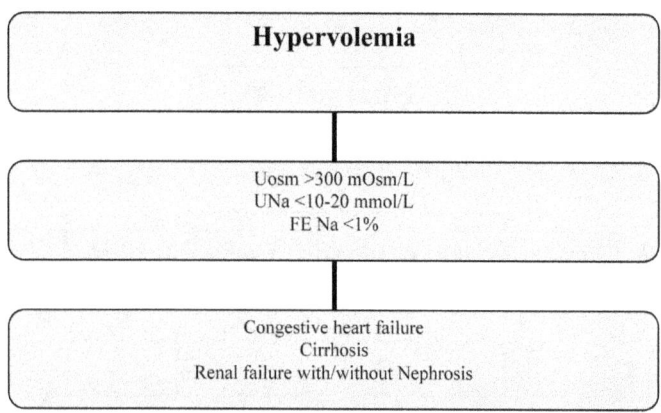

Hypernatremia (>145 mmol) occurs when water loss is in excess of salt loss; this can occur in severe diarrhea or vomiting and inadequate water intake. Hypernatremia also can be caused by diabetes insipidus.

Replacing the lost fluid with free water is the preferred treatment. If hemodynamically unstable, IV normal saline may be used until intravascular volume is corrected. Rapid and aggressive correction of serum sodium can lead to cerebral edema and neurologic injury. Correction of the sodium at a rate of 0.5 - 1 mmol/L per hour is recommended.

Determining water deficit

Corrected sodium = Na + (1.5 x (glucose-150)/100)
Water deficit = 0.6 x weight in kg x (sodium/140 - 1)

Hypocalcemia (<8.5 mg/dL; <2.12 mmol/L, ionized calcium <1 mmol/L) may be caused by dysfunction of the parathyroid or vitamin D system. Serum albumin must be considered in order to obtain an accurate assessment of the hypocalcemia.

Treatment is with IV calcium gluconate 1-2 g calcium given over 10 to 20 minutes followed by slow infusion at 0.5 to 1.5 mg/kg/hr.

Thyroid Test Interpretation

TSH	Free T4	Free T3	Interpretation
Normal	Normal	Normal	Thyroid disease excluded
Low	Normal	Low or normal	Non-thyroid illness vs. subclinical hyperthyroidism
Low	High	Low, high or normal	Non-thyroid illness vs. primary thyrotoxicosis
Low	Normal	High	T3 thyrotoxicosis
Low	Low	Low	Non-thyroid illness vs. central hypothyroidism
High	Low	Low or normal	Primary hypothyroidism
High or normal	High	High	Central hyperthyroidism

*"The art of medicine consists of amusing the patient
while nature cures the disease"*
Voltaire

9

Infectious Disease

Evaluation of fever in the ICU. The onset of fever in the critical care setting must be carefully evaluated clinically for the presence of new infection. Infection can arise through the use of invasive lines such as endotracheal tubes and urinary catheters. Surgical site infections may also cause fever as well and examination of recent medication additions should be made while looking for cause.

The choice to treat with antibiotics is made after careful consideration of the patient's clinical picture. If the patient's condition is life threatening, empiric antibiotics are given after cultures have been obtained. Definitive antibiotic therapy may be considered after the offending microorganism is identified.

Nosocomial infections should be considered if the patient has been hospitalized for over 72 hours, has been hospitalized in the last three months and has had multiple trials of antibiotics in the past.

Infections include:

Meningitis: Community acquired bacterial meningitis caused by S. pneumoniae or N. meningitidis. Treat with 3rd generation cephalosporins.

Community acquired pneumonia: Usually caused by S. pneumoniae but may be Legionella, Mycopasma or Chlamydia in origin. Treat with a B-lactam plus either a macrolide or fluoroquinolone.

Ventilator associated pneumonia (VAP): Caused by gram-negative microorganisms or S. aureus. Treat with a 3rd or 4th generation cephalosporin, B-lactam/B lactamase inhibitor. May also use a carbapenem plus a fluorqinolone or aminoglycoside.

Catheter related infections: Caused by coag-negative Staphylococcus or S. aureus. Treat with nafcillin. If MRSA in considered, treat with vancomycin. May also be caused by Candida, treat with fluconazole.

Urinary Tract Infection: Caused by Gram-negative enteric bacteria. Treat with 3rd generation cephalosporins, fluoroquinolones, aminoglycosides, piperacillin/ tazobactam or trimethoprim/sulfamethoxazole

Antibiotic-associated Colitis: Caused by C. difficile. Treat with metronidazole or vancomycin.

> *"It is health that is real wealth and*
> *not pieces of gold and silver"*
> *Mohandas Gandhi*

10
Fluids and Resuscitation

Fluid resuscitation is indicated when end organ perfusion is compromised. This is demonstrated by decreased intravascular pressure with a resultant decrease in urine output of less than 0.5mL/kg/hr. The type of fluid to be used is indicated by the cause of the problem.

Isotonic crystalloid solutions such as 0.9% saline and Lactated Ringer's add volume to the circulating blood volume. A fluid challenge of a large volume of crystalloid solution over a short period of time may be given to assess the patient's response to increased intravascular volume. Isotonic crystalloid solutions may also disperse into the interstitial space as well as to the lungs in prolonged fluid resuscitation.

Blood or blood components are indicated in the case of hemorrhage and is considered when total blood loss has been estimated to be greater than 30% of total blood volume (>1500 ml) and/or the Hgb is less that 7g/dL.

Colloids such as albumin and dextran may also be used to expand blood volume. These solutions may maintain plasma oncotic pressure more effectively than colloids.

For this reason, these should be avoided in trauma and traumatic brain injury patients.

General guideline for fluid resuscitation

Using crystalloid solution; for adults administer a 250-500 cc bolus, repeating as needed to maintain blood pressure and urine output of > 5ml/kg/hr.

Electrolyte Content of IV Solutions per Liter

Solution	Na	K	Glucose	Tonicity	mOsm/ liter
0.9 NS	154	0	0	Slightly hypertonic	304
0.45 NS	77	0	0	Hypotonic	154
0.25 NS	38	0	0	Hypotonic	77
Lactated Ringers	130	4	0	Isotonic	280
D5W	0	0	50gm	Hypotonic	0
D5W 0.45 NS	77	0	50gm	Hypotonic	154
0.9 NS + 150 mEq NaHCO3	308	0	0	Very Hypertonic	616

"The miserable have no other medicine but only hope"
William Shakespeare

11
Nutrition

Basal Metabolic Rate Formula

Men: BMR = (13.7516 x weight + 5.0033 x height - 6.755 x age + 66.473) kcal/day

Women: BMR = (9.5634 x weight + 1.8496 x height - 4.6756 x age + 655.0955) kcal/day

The Harris Benedict Equation is used to calculate the individual's predicted daily calorie expenditure. The equation uses the basal metabolic rate and multiplies by an activity factor in order to predict the daily calories needed to maintain the current weight.

Little to no exercise	BMR x 1.2
Light exercise	BMR x 1.375
Moderate exercise	BMR x 1.55
Heavy exercise	BMR x 1.725
Very heavy exercise	BMR x 1.9
Stress factor/hypermetabolism in critical illness	BMR x 1.1 - 2.0

Enteral Nutrition should be considered within 24-48 hours of the patient's admission to the critical care unit. Feeding the gut early has resulted in improved wound healing, preservation of the gastric mucosa and improved clinical outcomes.

Complications of enteral nutrition include high gastric residuals, bacterial colonization of the gut and increased risk for aspiration pneumonia.

Total Parenteral Nutrition is considered in cases where it is inadvisable to use the gut in a timely fashion for nutrition needs. TPN preparations include amino acids, carbohydrates, lipids, electrolytes, MVI and minerals. TPN must be infused using a central venous catheter.

Other nutritional requirements include:

Protein: 1.0 to 1.8 grams protein/kg per day

Lipids: 30 to 70 grams /day

Other calorie sources:

Propofol provides 1 cal/ml of product.

Peritoneal dialysis or CAVHD - 35-45% of administered dextrose is absorbed.

"[It] is easy, as we can see, for a barbarian to be healthy;
for a civilized man the task is hard."
Sigmund Freud

www.ingramcontent.com/pod-product-compliance
Lightning Source LLC
Chambersburg PA
CBHW051245170526
45165CB00004B/1579